Rewrite Your Life Without Dermatographia

Rewrite *your*
LIFE
WITHOUT
Dermatographia

The All-Natural Solution to Managing
Hive-like Welts & Severe Itching

SANDRA GRANEAU

NEW YORK

LONDON • NASHVILLE • MELBOURNE • VANCOUVER

Rewrite Your Life Without Dermatographia

The All-Natural Solution to Managing Hive-like Welts and Severe Itching

© 2020 Sandra Graneau

Published in New York, New York, by Morgan James Publishing in partnership with Difference Press. Morgan James is a trademark of Morgan James, LLC. www.MorganJamesPublishing.com

ISBN 9781642794755 paperback
ISBN 9781642794762 eBook
ISBN 9781642795608 audiobook
Library of Congress Control Number: 2019901297

Cover & Interior Design by:
Christopher Kirk
www.GFSstudio.com

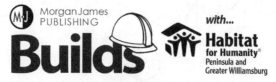

Morgan James is a proud partner of Habitat for Humanity Peninsula and Greater Williamsburg. Partners in building since 2006.

Get involved today! Visit
MorganJamesPublishing.com/giving-back

For those of you who have big dreams that scare you.
Despite life's challenges, you keep striving
to make your dreams come true anyways.
I salute you. Never give up.

Table of Contents

Introduction:
When the Writing is Not on the Wall

If you are picking up this book to review or read it, it's because you have dermatographia, know someone who has it, or you are just curious because you've never heard of this skin condition.

First, a little disclaimer: I am not a doctor, healthcare provider, or claim to be a healer. All the information presented is used for informational purpose only. It is not intended to replace the medical advice of your doctor or healthcare provider. Please consult with your doctor first for advice about your condition.

There is an idiom that you may have heard mentioned as "The writing was on the wall." It means that there was a warning that failure or disaster was on its way before the actual event took place.

But what happens when the writing is on your skin? When you must always be careful about what touches your body? Scratching your skin causes it to turn red and creates welts, but you can't help it because the itchiness is intense. The remaining marks can stay on your skin for 30 minutes or last a whole day. Your skin is so sensitive that you can lightly write your name and within seconds your skin will elevate and show your name in 3D. Is this a warning of something else going on? If so, what is happening? This skin condition is called dermatographia.

Dermatographia is also known as dermatographism, and dermographic urticaria. Most online resources of information for dermatographia give similar descriptions of the condition. Here is one from healthline.com:

"Dermatographia, which is sometimes called "skin writing," refers to a condition in which seemingly minor scratches turn into temporary but significant reactions. This condition is also called dermographism or dermatographic urticaria. Approximately five percent of people have this condition..."

Although symptoms vary for each person, they may include:
- Redness
- Red raised marks on the skin that look like writing
- Deep wounds
- Hive-like welts
- Itchiness
- Swelling or inflammation

Symptoms can last about 30 minutes or in severe cases, last a day or more. Dermographia itself can last for months – or even years – and there is no cure. Its exact cause is unknown. According to the Cleveland Clinic website:

"Dermatograhismis most likely caused by an inappropriate release of histamine in the absence of a typical immune signal. The red welts and hives are caused by the local effect of histamine."

Other causes include:

- Stress
- Heat or Cold Exposure
- Exercise
- Vibration
- A history of allergies
- Excessive rubbing from clothing or bedding
- Infections
- Certain medications
- Alcohol

The first time you dealt with a symptom of dermatographia, your reaction may have been nonchalant. You may have thought, "Oh, my hands may be dry. I need to put some more lotion on." When you saw your first welt you may have asked, "Did I walk into something by accident and don't remember?" or "Maybe my clothes were too tight, that may have caused a welt. I will make sure I don't wear my belt so snug again."

However, when you started to notice the scratches and welts appeared more often, you became a little bit more concerned. You know you moisturized your skin very well, you didn't walk into anything, and your clothes are not tight on you, but the itchiness, the redness, and welts continued to appear. The interesting thing is that depending on what is happening in your life, these symptoms do not appear regularly. They show up intermittently.

First, you may think you are allergic to the lotion or the material that your clothes are made of. So you stop using the lotion or wearing clothes made with certain materials. You may even go as far to change your diet – cut out dairy and red meat, minimize the amount of bread you eat or avoid gluten or stop eating onions and garlic. You probably think this is happening because you are low in a vitamin or mineral, so you increase your supplemental vitamin intake. However, the symptoms still appear.

You may not be able to find out the exact thing that is causing the symptoms to appear, but they are now showing up frequently and more consistently in certain areas. Now you start to pay attention to everything you touch and eat. You begin to feel confused and overwhelmed by what is happening to you. You may start thinking about any past or childhood history of these symptoms. You may ask your parent if they recall you having certain childhood skin conditions or breakouts.

You will go on the internet to research if anyone else is suffering from these symptoms and what they have done to ease their condition. You may try multiple suggestions, only to find out their suggestions do not work out for you as you would have liked. At this point, you feel like you want to jump out of your skin. You start to think about seeing your doctor, but how do you explain your experience without coming across as weird or crazy? Will your doctor even know what you're talking about? A sense of hopelessness may rush over you.

You take a chance and visit your doctor. You try to explain the symptoms, hoping you do not seem like you're making things up and when you try to scratch yourself to show the welts, nothing happens. How convenient! It's like telling the I.T. person at work the problems you're having with company's software but the moment they show up and touch the computer, it works fine.

All of this is emotionally draining. You do not understand what is really going on, how it all began, and how to stop it. The itchiness is unbearable, and the welts and redness are unsightly. If the symptoms appear in public, people may think you are injuring yourself or you are a freak. The emotional toll is too heavy to bear, and you wish there was someone who could tell you what is going on and understand the overwhelming sense of helplessness you feel.

Now you may feel like you are alone in this situation, and you may fear rejection. Who will understand what you're going through? Will they make fun of your condition? If they knew what you are dealing with will they still like you? When people see your welts and redness, will they understand that you are not intentionally hurting yourself? These questions and other thoughts may arise, causing you to feel isolated or want to isolate yourself. Please know for a fact that dermatographia is real. You are not alone.

Chapter 1:
The Itch

There is a saying that if the palm of your right-hand itches, then money is coming your way. If the palm of your left-hand itches, then you are going to lose money. What happens if both palms are itching? Nothing? Not necessarily.

If you have itchy palms and other symptoms of dermatographia, it does not matter what an old wives' tale says. Aside from the emotional toll dermatographia may have on you, it can be costly in other areas in your life. Doctor visits, purchasing medications, finances, relationships, your body and confidence my pay the price for dermatographia.

If you have a doctor to whom you've explained your symptoms and he or she was able to recognize the signs of dermatographia on your first visit, you are fortunate. Many people must visit more than one doctor to get the correct diagnosis. The time it takes to drive to the doctor's office and pay deductibles and co-pays costs time and money.

Once you find a doctor or specialist who understands the symptoms you're experiencing, they may ask you to take a skin and/or allergy test. If the test(s) confirms what you've been trying to articulate, based on the results you may receive the diagnosis of dermatographia. After you've received your diagnosis, the doctor or specialist may tell you to purchase an over-the-counter medication to help minimize the symptoms. They might consult with you on what you should avoid or suggest products you may try to help soothe the reactions of dermatographia. The tests, over-the-counter medications, bathing products, purchasing of new clothes to accommodate your condition, and whatever else you may have bought, costs money.

Now you've received the diagnosis of dermatographia, you realize that since there is no cure and you do not know how long you may have to live with this condition, you may have to revamp your lifestyle. The money you would have liked to save for the future or for vacation is being spent on minimizing your symptoms of dermatographia.

What about the cost this skin condition is having on your relationships? Does your significant other, family, and/or close friends know about your dermatographia? If they do, how did they react? Did they jump back if you showed them the reaction your skin makes when you scratch or put a little pressure on it? Did they ask you if you're contagious? Did you receive any other adverse reactions when you tried to explain your symptoms? Did they empathize with you and ask what they could do to help? Did you have to change the way you held each other? Are you afraid of getting into an intimate relationship because of it?

All these reactions and more are possible from the special people in your life. Hopefully they approached the situation with love and understanding. However, they may need to adjust to your new lifestyle as well and change how they interact with you to avoid aggravating your symptoms. This is a cost.

The knowledge of your diagnosis can add additional stress on your body. You are feeling overwhelmed by all the changes. Now you may be overly sensitive to how you hold things to or on your body. You may wear your clothes differently to avoid prolonged welts that may cause scarring on the skin. Your skin may be extremely sensitive to touch and temperatures. All the scratching you've been doing may make your skin feel like it's burning. You may have to change your diet to help control your symptoms. The stress of trying to do the best you can to ease your skin condition, is a cost your body is paying.

The final price may come in the form of your confidence. Whether or not you have high or low confidence prior to finding out about your condition, your confidence will take a hit. The thought of having dermatographia for months, years, or a lifetime may inspire a lot of questions. Why me? How did this all start? What can I do to change this? How do I live with this condition without making others uncomfortable? Can someone really love me if they find out I have dermatographia? Will I have to constantly wear pants and long sleeve shirts to avoid people from staring at me if they see my symptoms? Will they see me as a person, or will they just see my symptoms? Can all of this just stop? These are a few questions that you may have asked. Doubts can cause your confidence to decrease.

Dermatographia may also impact your confidence at work. Since you are already self-conscious of reactions happening and symptoms may arise while you're at your job, it may be difficult for you to focus on assignments or projects. The lack of focus may come across to your coworkers or boss as a lack of dedication. Since doubt is already on your mind about the impact of your skin condition and you think your peers and boss at work think that you're easily distracted, you may not feel you're capable of getting the next promotion or opportunity.

What I presented are just examples of how dermatographia is costing you. You may have other experiences not mentioned in this chapter, but overall no matter what it is, there is a cost of living with dermatographia and its impact in all aspects of your life.

This book will show you how you can live your life freely without being concerned about dermatographia. In the following chapters, I will share my story with dermatographia. You will learn the process of dealing with the reality of the condition, the possible triggers for your symptoms, the tools you need to overcome your triggers, and how to find the right people to help you through the process and set boundaries. Finally, you'll learn to navigate your life to avoid reoccurrences and what to do when there is a setback.

Chapter 2:

My Story

Istarted to get symptoms of dermatographia four years ago. I was working multiple jobs and I started my own book-keeping service. During the day, I would go to the office to work. At night, I would come home to complete work for my clients. Aside from work, I also had a few personal projects going on. I planned my life to be busy nearly every hour of the day with enough time to sleep for eight hours. Not a minute was wasted.

One night, I noticed an itchiness in the palm of my right hand. Of course I thought, "Oh, money is coming to me very soon." I chalked it up to dry skin and I put lotion on my hands. The itchiness occurred again another night. I thought my hand was itching because my lotion wasn't strong enough, so I started using coconut oil. Then the palm of my left hand started to itch around the same time my right palm would itch. I became confused and looked on the internet what would cause itchy palms. Most of the information encountered was about dry, chafed skin. I made sure that my hands – especially my palms – were extremely moisturized.

Pretty soon the bottoms of my feet started to itch. It was unbearable. My feet would itch shortly after the palms of my hands stopped itching. I felt something was wrong, but although the episodes would be intense, they were short and seemingly random. After an episode, the palms of my hands and the bottom of my feet would be beet red. Occasionally it was so intense I used to use a ruler or a letter opener to apply pressure into my hands and feet while I scratched, because the itch felt like it was below the surface of my hands and feet. The funny thing was that these episodes only occurred at night while I was working.

It wasn't until I saw my first welt that I realized I may be dealing with something serious. I was changing my clothes after work when I noticed a long welt along my stomach where my belt was located. Because I use to have skin outbreaks as a kid, I thought maybe I was experiencing a childhood skin outbreak. But then the welt around my waist continued to appear every night. After an hour, it would disappear. I started to wear tanks and T-shirts under my work clothes so my jeans and belt would not touch my skin. Constant welts around my waist started to leave a mark on my skin when they would fade away. Throughout this time, I did not associate the itchiness in my hand and feet to the welts on my stomach.

I knew I had a physical exam coming up. I decided I was going to talk to my doctor about the symptoms I was experiencing. On my visit, I tried to explain what I was going through on my stomach and showed the scar line on my waist. By this time, I'd learned to layer clothes to minimize the welts. The doctor did not seem to know what I was talking about. I left the office without a solution.

Shortly afterward, I started to see large welt marks around my breast from my bras. Not only did my hands and feet itch regularly, and my waist was welting, but my whole chest area where my bras were fitted snugly to my skin were causing large welt marks. Sometimes it would be painful to take off my bra, because the swelling from the welt was so intense. There were occasions when it was so bad that when air touched my skin it would burn.

I started to think I was allergic to something I was eating. I began to change my diet – no dairy, no meat, and no bread. I thought over time my symptoms would go away. They didn't. All of them appeared regularly and intensity increased.

One day during my day job, I was preparing for a presentation and I had a large stack of papers in my arms. I was wearing a short-sleeve top. I completed putting all the papers together for my presentation and was stacking the binders when I looked down at my arms. Both of my forearms were red with numerous welts that looked like slashes. This was a new location for my symptom.

The visual of numerous slash-looking welts on my forearms gave me the chills. I was scared. Fortunately, I had a sweater to cover my arms during the presentation. A couple hours later, I checked my arms and it seemed that like nothing ever happened in the first place. When I had another paper-related episode on my arms, I made an appointment with an allergist's office.

I went and explained what I was experiencing. The specialist scratched my arm, but nothing happened. Just great! He agreed to let me take an allergy test. I took the test and left. I went into my car and cried. I knew I was not crazy. There was something going on in my body that I did not understand and I could not stop it. None of the symptoms were showing up for the doctors, so it seemed like I didn't know what I was talking about.

As I waited for the results to validate what I was experiencing, the symptoms continued. The doctor called me with the results. I tested negative for all possible allergies. They said I was not allergic to anything. I couldn't believe it. What was happening? The symptoms were not stopping, and I could barely focus on my work because of the episodes.

I documented my outbreaks by taking pictures of my skin whenever welts would appear and I made another appointment with the allergy specialist. I told him although my results said I didn't have any allergies, something was going on with my body. I showed him the pictures and explained my symptoms again. Immediately, he told me I had dermatographic urticaria, a form of hives.

I told him that I had been dealing with this for over a year. He said that he could not tell how much longer I would have to deal with the symptoms, and that there was no cure for this skin condition. He suggested that I make a change in my lifestyle to minimize my stress and that I take Loratadine or Benadryl to help minimize the symptoms.

When I left the office, I was overwhelmed. I bought the medications, but they didn't help. My symptoms seemed to get stronger even though I took the pills as directed. I realized if the pills were not working and my diet wasn't the issue, then I needed to make changes to my lifestyle. Being faced with a condition that can be debilitating at times made me reevaluate everything in my life. I began to think about how my life would be if I had a chance to do things over. What I came up with was this: I was sick and tired of how I had been living for the last two years, and I wanted my symptoms to go away once and for all.

I decided to act on the doctor's advice. The first thing I did was let go of my day job and the multiple side projects. I decided to put all of my focus on my business. I started a year-long life coach training. I also had a revelation that the trauma from my past was contributing to my symptoms, so I went to see a therapist. To help me get physically healthy, I hired a personal trainer to get me back on track with exercising.

Within one year I noticed the intensity of my symptoms had started to decrease. I stopped taking Loratadine and Benadryl. A few months later, I started taking acting classes and sketching hanboks (Korean traditional clothes) for fun. I noticed when I was participating in these two activities, I felt like a child or like time did not exist. My welts stopped appearing as often.

As time passed, I started to become conscious of who I had in my circle. I surrounded myself with people who wanted the best for me. I recognized that I needed to leave a couple of toxic relationships and to set boundaries. By that time, the itchiness in my hands and feet barely occurred.

I decided that I was going to treat myself as my most valuable asset. I continued to work out, I made "me days" just to relax, and I tried my best to get enough rest so I could be clear-minded the next day. I didn't share my experience with everyone;

only a select few, and mostly with God. Since I've been training to be a life coach, I would ask myself hard questions that challenged my beliefs and made me change my perspectives on my past and my present. I made a decision to commit to creating the life I wanted to live. For the last two years, I have been symptom free from dermatographia.

Chapter 3:

The Process

There's one solution to having a life without being concerned about dermatographia: make a decision. That's it. Even if you don't feel like it, make the decision that you are worth the commitment to make the necessary changes so dermatographia is not controlling your life. Be willing to make the investment in yourself to find the right people who will help you create a new perspective, new ideas, and move forward in the direction you want your life to be. Trust yourself that you are strong enough to handle the emotional pain you must face while you are going through this process. You must be willing to do the work I'm leading you through. So make a decision.

In this book, you will find out the root problem(s) of your symptoms' triggers, and learn physical, mental and spiritual tools to assist you to obtain a balance in your life. You will understand how people can make a big impact in your life and to know when to get out of a toxic relationship and set boundaries. Finally, you will learn how to navigate your life to avoid reoccurrence of dermatographia and what to do when "life happens."

No one is going to make you do anything you do not want to do. You can read this book, appreciate the information, take notes, and then add it to your bookshelf. At this stage, it's normal for you to wonder if reading a book will minimize your dermatographia.

Take Mindy's example. Mindy has had dermatographia for many years. She has read all the self-help books and online blogs/articles, takes medication for relief from her symptoms, changed her diet and has a lifestyle that helps her cope with dermatographia. However, she continues to have dermatographic episodes. Mindy is so emotionally drained that she is quietly asking for help within her spirit. She heard of my experience with dermatographia and asked for coaching sessions. When it came time to deal with her emotional pain, Mindy shut down. She didn't want to go "there." It would be too much work.

When I asked Mindy what she meant, she explained that she was scared what her life would be like without dermatographia. She had had it for so long, that she had become to identify herself by this skin disorder. What would happen to everything she knew if things would change? I asked her, "What will continue to happen if you do not change? What is your current lifestyle costing you with dermatographia?"

Mindy took a long pause to think about these questions. After we discussed the pros and cons, she realized that to continue to live with dermatographia would cost her a lot more than what she had to lose if she took the leap of faith. When Mindy overcame her identity block, she was able to excel in the process and overcome dermatographia.

To succeed in this process, you must be dedicated to make it work and disciplined in changing how you think and talk about and to yourself. While you are reading this book, use what resonates with you. You may have different root issues for your triggers and symptoms, all of which is valid. Use the process as a framework to get you the life you want, a life free without being concerned or affected by dermatographia.

Chapter 4:
Fireworks

Our bodies are amazing machines. For the most part, your body will do whatever it can to repair itself. It also sends you messages when something isn't working right or is out of place. This is what we call dis-ease or dis-ease. Usually we go to the doctor, find out what is wrong, take the medication prescribed to us, and, if it is not a serious illness, we go back home and hope whatever we are going through will correct itself so we can get back to our normal life.

However, outside of hereditary diseases, certain causes of dis-ease may be rooted in our past, our current disappointments, or internal fears. Certain triggers or circumstances in our present can send us reeling back to traumatic childhood experiences, remind us of our failures, or confirm our worst fears.

Medical or health websites may list the causes for dermatographia, but what we want to do is find out the top triggers behind those causes. The listed causes in the introduction of this book are really the symptoms of a deeper situation. As I stated before, certain actions or situations can trigger your symptoms. According to an article from Medical News Today:

"Triggers can include heat, activity, and emotional circumstances. For example, 44 percent of participants in one study said stress could cause acute episodes of skin writing."

In this chapter, I am going to focus on the triggers of stress connected to emotional pain and physical activity.

Stress is your body's reaction to harmful situations that are real or perceived. This reaction is known as "fight-or-flight." Each person handles stress differently. Some people can handle it very well and use it to accomplish goals. Others may physically or mentally shut down when there is too much stress. Your body is capable of handling a small amount of stress over time, but continuous stress can start manifesting into various symptoms. The symptoms of stress can be emotional, physical, mental, and behavioral.

Emotional symptoms can include the following: depression, low self-esteem, constant worrying, feeling the need to take control or lose control, being frustrated or moody, and being disappointed in yourself.

Emotional pain can trigger symptoms of dermatographia. Here are some examples of situations that can cause emotional pain:

Relationships: being in a toxic relationship, having a cheating partner, dealing with a divorce and/or custody battle.

Take Mary. Mary took pride in her marriage. She loved her husband, and had two wonderful girls in college. To help with the transition of empty nesting, Mary asked her husband if he could take time off from work so they could start traveling as a couple. He told her that he would work on it and for her to go ahead and plan their trip.

Two weeks later, she finished planning the trip and met with her husband in the kitchen. She kept talking about how excited she was and did not notice a letter on the kitchen counter in front of her husband. When she was done, she noticed the letter and asked her husband what it was. He said, "Mary, I want a divorce." Mary felt like the air was kicked out of her body, as she stood in shock.

In the next several days as Mary tried to figure out what went wrong in her marriage, what she did wrong, and how she missed the signs, her body started to itch. She noticed several times that whenever she scratched her skin, welts would appear. The emotional pain from the loss of her marriage caused Mary to have episodes of dermatographia.

Another emotional trigger could be family. Whether it be caused by physical, mental, or sexual abuse, a death of family member, a strained communication with family members, abandonment, betrayal, or rejection from family members, family is a large part of our lives that could easily trigger your symptoms.

For example, Peter had strained relationship with his father. Although he would see his father almost every night when he came home from work, his father seemed disinterested in what was going on in Peter's life. This wasn't a surprise; in school, Peter had enjoyed performing musical theater. Whenever he had a performance, he asked his father if he could attend the show. His father never came to any of his performances.

One day, Peter was awarded the lead role in a popular musical theater show. He hoped that if he told his father the great news the night before the show opening and provided him a ticket, maybe his father would show up to this performance. Peter bought the ticket, told his father about winning the lead role, and the time of the show. He presented the ticket to his father. His father looked at him for a moment, looked at the ticket on the table, and then got up and walked away without taking the ticket or saying a word.

Peter was devastated by the rejection. He decided to use the energy for his performance. Although he received a standing ovation for his performance the opening night, it didn't feel fulfilling without his father present. While he was taking off his costume, Peter noticed red welts across his chest where the costume was rubbing against his skin.

The next emotional trigger can be personal, such as having low self-esteem, being self-critical, self-hatred, depression, feeling like a victim, or being judgmental of others. It can also come from being disappointed in your life choices, unsatisfied with your accomplishments, and by setting extremely high standards that even you cannot achieve.

Take Joanne, who was always a stellar student. She maintained a 4.0 GPA in high school and through her first two years in college. When her mother lost her job, Joanne decided to get a job to help with expenses. As she began to work, she lost the time she usually took to study. She noticed that she was struggling to maintain an "A" in one of her classes. This concerned Joanne and she began to doubt her abilities as a student.

Soon Joanne started to listen to the critical voices in her head that she wouldn't amount to anything because she couldn't maintain straight "As" in all her class. Joanne started to stress about her situation. She struggled to study with time she didn't have. She couldn't quit her job, because her family needed the money. She knew that she wasn't going to drop out of school – that wasn't an option she would consider.

Joanne felt overwhelmed and disappointed in herself for the situation she was in. One day after studying, she noticed red lines on her legs where her books were resting on her lap. The lines freaked her out and confused her when they didn't go away immediately. When she looked at her legs again 45 minutes later, the lines were gone, and her legs appeared as though nothing happened.

Physical symptoms are also a trigger, and can be classified by aches and tense muscles, upset stomach, insomnia, colds and infections, nervousness, dry mouth, low or no energy, headaches or migraines, clenched teeth, chest pain, or rapid heartbeat.

Suzanne exemplifies these symptoms. She won a major project at work. She was excited for the future opportunities that would arise if she exceeded expectations upon completion of the project. Midway through the project, Suzanne's boyfriend became seriously ill and was hospitalized. Since he did not have any family in town, Suzanne would make trips to the hospital with her available time.

Soon, Suzanne became sick with a cold. She didn't want to take time off from work, because that would cause her to be late on her deadline. In her off time, instead of going to the hospital to visit her boyfriend, she would go home to lay down and work remotely. The more she kept pushing herself to work, the sicker she became. Eventually, her boss told her to take a couple of days off to rest and get better. In her absence, the project would be handled by someone else. Suzanne was not happy about the situation but understood that the stress she was feeling from her desire of wanting to exceed expectations and her boyfriend's illness was making her ill.

The second to last type of trigger can be mental symptoms. These can be forgetfulness, lack of focus, bad judgment, constant worrying, non-stop thoughts, and viewing the world from a negative perspective.

Jerry was running late for work again. In the last few weeks since Jerry's promotion to upper management, he had been dealing with the worry of "am I good enough." He wondered if he took more than he could handle. This worry had caused Jerry to begin to doubt his decisions when he dealt with employees. He noticed that he couldn't seem to remember where he placed things, especially his keys. Ironically, each time he couldn't find his keys to get to work on time, it was a day he had a business meeting with a client. Jerry noticed the stress of his worry, doubts, and the responsibilities of his work impacted him mentally.

Finally, behavioral symptoms are a major potential trigger. Behavioral symptoms can be classified as procrastination, changes in how you eat, avoiding responsibilities, increase in drug or alcohol intake, and nervous behaviors like nail biting, pacing, and fidgeting.

An example of this would be Naomi, who needed to take her son to the doctor for the completion of his school medical form before the beginning of the school year. Since there were still two months before school started, Naomi decided that she would schedule the doctor's appointment after their vacation.

When Naomi and her son returned from vacation, she remembered that she needed to make the appointment for her son's doctor, but decided to wait until three weeks before school started. The week of the first day of school, Naomi was rushing to get everything she needed to get for her son. She realized that she forgot to make the appointment for the doctor. When she called to make the appointment, the next available appointment was one week after school started.

Since Naomi couldn't wait that long, she took her son to an urgent care center to be seen by another doctor, so her son could go to school on time. Naomi realized her procrastination was not only costing her time, but it also affected her son's life.

Based on the number of symptoms listed for stress, it is not surprising that stress is the highest contributor of outbreaks of dermatographia.

On the other hand, physical activity can be a potential trigger. Physical activity can be considered structured exercise like playing sports, or more normal activities such as playing with your kids at the park or beach, cleaning your house, taking an extended walk outside, taking a vacation, or taking the subway to and from work daily can constitute as physical activities. Each of these examples may increase your body heat or cause constant friction to the body, which can aggravate or trigger dermatographia.

Julia liked to spend quiet time in her garden during the day. The time she spent amongst her flowers and plants was relaxing. If it got too hot and Julia started sweating, she wrapped up her gardening and went inside. When she changed, Julia always checked her legs to see if she had a dermatographia outbreak. She noticed that if she stayed outside too long in the heat, an episode would occur between her inner thighs from the friction of being on her hands and knees while gardening.

Usually when we think of activity, we only think about physical activity. However, activity can also be working long hours without taking enough time for rest. It can be constantly worrying about situations without letting them go. It can also be when you try to control your life and not release yourself to your spiritual beliefs. If you do not allow yourself to rest physically, mentally, or spiritually, these can be triggers for your symptoms.

Since high school, Sophia had a list of all that she wanted to accomplish in her life. She knew what college she wanted to attend, the type of career she wanted to excel in, the man she wanted to marry, the type of house in a certain location she would like to have, and number of children.

Everything on her list, Sophia was able to achieve. The only thing that was missing was children. After ten years of marriage, Sophia and her husband were unsuccessful in getting pregnant. They decided to try in vitro fertilization. IVF is an expensive process and put a strain on her body, their finances, and their relationship.

Emotionally, Sophia was starting to wear down and began to blame God and herself for not being able to have children. Her dermatographia returned with intensity. She knew that she needed to get rest, but Sophia was completely drained physically, emotionally, and spiritually. She was restless and felt like she was at a loss.

Can you relate to any of these stories? If so, it is time to recognize and acknowledge that stress, lack of rest, or emotional pain may be contributing to your dermatographia. Being aware that the decisions you've made, the circumstance in your life, and how you treat yourself are contributing to your dermatographia is very scary. As you process it, it can feel overwhelming to know that you have a choice to make a change.

Changing means leaving what is familiar to you. It means that you are taking the risk to walk into the unknown, to have faith in the future, to learn to unlearn bad habits and relearn new ones. Some changes can be made right away. Some may take months or years. Changes may cost you a relationship or money. However, deciding right now to make a change to not continue to live your life being controlled by dermatographia takes bravery and you are brave enough to do it.

Chapter 5:

Can You Pass Me the Hammer?

So, you made the decision to make a change. What's next? Take a deep breath. Congratulations on making this big decision! Now we are going to review a couple of physical, mental, and spiritual tools that you can start using in your daily life. Keep in mind, you do not need to do everything at one time. You just made a big shift. Start with one thing at a time and build from there.

The first tool is physical exercise. Physical exercise is necessary for our bodies to be at its best. For most people it is a stress reliever. According to the American Heart Association, for overall cardiovascular health and lowering blood pressure and cholesterol, their recommendation is at least 30 minutes of moderate- to vigorous-intensity aerobic exercise at least three times per week.

You can go to the gym, work out at home, or take a walk in your neighborhood. Find out what environment works best for you. If going to the gym is too intimidating or distracting, then don't go there. Try another alternative. Working out at home may be less expensive and convenient for you. If working out at home makes you long for your couch every thirty seconds or you get easily distracted, try something else.

Taking an early morning or sunset walk at a nearby park or school track may work for you. Gardening or spring cleaning your home can be a form of exercise. You may be someone who likes to participate in activity with others. If so, you can consider a sport that you're interested in, dancing classes, workout at home with family members or playing with your kids. If exercise is a trigger for your dermatographia, consider changing your routine or consider another form of exercise that may not agitate your symptoms.

The point is that you do not have to do what everyone else does or what you think you're supposed to do. Find a physical activity that works with your schedule and your finances, and that you can consistently continue. If you struggle to start the workout you've scheduled, it could be that you're tired or that exercise is not the right fit for you. After your workout, you should have a surge of energy and a sense of accomplishment.

If you find out your workout clothes may aggravate your dermatographia symptoms, try loose or cotton clothing when you work out. Loose clothing and cotton material will allow your skin to breathe and minimize irritation to your skin.

For example, Jennifer wore form-fitting workout clothes. She liked to use the stair climber during her workout. She went to the doctor because she noticed welts were showing up on her legs and chest where the seams of her work-out clothes rubbed against her skin. Her doctor suggested that she tried more loose-fitting workout clothes. Jennifer took his advice and wore the new clothes at the gym. After her workout, she noticed that the welts did not appear on her legs and were less prevalent on her chest.

Before starting any exercise regimen, check with your doctor to find out if it is safe to continue the workout you are interested in.

Improving your diet is another tool that you can use to improve your symptoms. Most of the time when we eat, we eat what we have an emotional connection to. Fast food is a go-to for lunches or last-minute meals. We eat out with friends and associates for dinners. Food has become a social connection.

We are fortunate to know several options in the grocery store to accommodate our needs. If you cannot drink dairy, there are soy, coconut, and almond milks available. Can't have gluten? There are gluten-free products available. There are organic produce and products, cage-free eggs, and grass-fed meat. Want your pick of sugar? There's white, brown, cane, raw, agave, stevia, etc. You will find anything you need to fit your dietary needs.

Before you make a change in your diet, take notes of everything you eat for a week. You can use an app for food logging or you can take pictures of your meals. After the week, review everything that you've eaten. Take one item (it can be more if you're up to it) that you noticed you eat the most that is not produce or a protein. You can switch the item for something else healthier or eliminate it from your diet the following week. Continue this method until you find yourself having the right diet that works for you.

Mike had dermatographia for several months. He decided to make changes to his diet. He wrote down everything he ate and then on a weekly basis removed or exchanged items in his diet to find out what was triggering his dermatographia. After two months, Mike found out that red meat and sugar triggered his dermatographia. He removed those two items, and nearly eliminated his dermatographia episodes. As a bonus, Mike lost twenty pounds in three months.

Depending on how severe your case of dermatographia is, another set of tools that you can practice that can be physically and mentally relaxing (if you stay in the moment) are massages, facials, or stretches. If you are comfortable with allowing a professional to touch you, massages or stretches allow the practitioner to work with your muscles in your body to release tension and toxins from your body. In a facial, not only are your pores cleaned, but your face is massaged to relax the muscles in your face. Most appointments are usually one-hour sessions.

This an opportunity to make "me time." During your session, release the thoughts about what you must do next and what you've forgotten to complete. Be present. Everything else can wait. When you are done with your session, you should feel relaxed and refreshed.

When you are looking for a place of business that provide massages, facials, or stretches, make sure you research the place online for good reviews or ask trusted friends and family for recommendations. You can also try your local beauty schools for services, their senior students need to practice for a certain number of hours in order to obtain their certification. The schools usually offer their services almost half the price a professional would normally charge.

I mentioned that massages, facials, or stretching can be mentally relaxing, but another mental tool that is underrated is rest. I am not talking about sleep. I am talking about getting rest.

Yes, we need to sleep for our brain to process the day and reboot itself for the next day. Without sleep we will die. Going to bed with a lot on your mind and looking at the clock tick on, is not rest. The definition for rest that I am talking about is freedom from activity or labor and peace of mind or spirit.

If your life is your work, freedom from activity or labor may be taking a long overdue vacation without making business calls or checking your work email while you are away from the office. It can be not allowing yourself to work every weekend or bring work home in the evening. It can also be organizing your desk, so the mess on it doesn't overwhelm you. The organized space will allow you to think clearly and minimize stress.

Being busy doesn't mean that you're productive. If you are someone who feels the need to have multiple things going on at the same time, yes, you are busy; but do you feel like you're accomplishing anything, or do you feel exhausted because you can't keep up? Are you someone who must have things perfect, that it is a challenge to let go of your control and delegate or share your responsibilities? At the end of the day, you wonder why you feel burdened by the weight of all the things you have to complete and feel like there's no one to help you.

Michelle was a mid-level manager who manages a team of seven. She struggled with getting her team on board to meet their monthly quotas and had a high turnover rate. Michelle felt frustrated that she could not maintain employees who were able to meet her expectations. Whenever a member of their team did not complete an assignment, Michelle would get frustrated and start micromanaging the employee. If a new hire started, she would provide the employee with a handbook and a couple of training sessions. After the training was completed, she didn't follow up with the employee until a mistake had been made.

Aside from her employees, Michelle had her own responsibilities as a manager. She needed help, but would not delegate duties, because she didn't believe that others could produce their work at the level she expected. This had caused her to work six days a week. Sometimes on her day off, she worked remotely just to be current on her emails. When she woke up in the morning, the first thing she thought about was what needed to be done at work. Sometimes she couldn't sleep because of the all the things that were running through her mind that needed to be accomplished.

The HR department called Michelle to their office. They notified her that they were receiving complaints from the employees. The complaints were her lack of availability for her team, insufficient training, and follow-up on how the employee was progressing, micromanaging, and the tense environment around her. Michelle was shocked and offended by what she heard. HR asked if she was willing to work on improving her relationship with her employees. Michelle felt at a loss. She didn't feel comfortable making a change because what she had done in the past worked for her. Michelle realized that what she was feeling was a loss of control.

The sense of being in control is an illusion that you can manipulate the circumstances around you to fit your comfort. Being in control only pushes away what you really want from you. If you cannot let go of your work, the projects or the multiple activities for a moment, a few hours or days, you do not have freedom. Although I used work as an example, these scenarios can be applied to other areas in your life. Until you can make designated time for yourself and release your control, you will not rest.

Rest as peace of mind and spirit, is when you are not filled with thoughts of worry, and blame. These emotions will rob you of your peace of mind. Constant worrying about situations going on in your life, whether they have occurred, or you are anticipating them, will make you restless. Worrying can also keep you awake at night when you need to sleep. One suggestion to help with running thoughts is to have a notepad or journal next to your bed. You can write down your thoughts down to release that energy from your body. If you are comfortable with cameras, you can also try to create a video journal of your thoughts with your smartphone or tablet.

Blame is thought of as holding someone or something else responsible for your status in life. I believe that it is a part of the victim mentality. Blame has a way of giving your mind permission to keep playing rewind to the story. To your mind, the events are still real. Allowing someone or something to have that kind of power over you will keep you stagnant in your current circumstance. Blame is also an excuse to justify why you can't improve your situation. If you want to make a change and you need to move forward in your life, you must release the blame you are carrying. Release the negative energy that is wearing you out. If the story of your blame is centered around a trauma, I would recommend that you find a licensed therapist who can assist you to process the circumstance that you've experienced.

Glen could only maintain a relationship for two years. Toward the end of the two years, Glen started flaking on dates, causing arguments about the littlest things, and taking other actions that would sabotage his relationships. Then he ghosts his partners.

When Glen was asked why he could not keep a long-term relationship, he blamed his mother for his abandonment issues. Glen couldn't get over the experience of his mother dropping him off at his friend's birthday party at the age of six, and never returning to get him. Glen held a subconscious belief that if he stayed with someone for a long period of time and became emotionally attached to her, she would leave him eventually. Before his girlfriend had the opportunity to "abandon" Glen, he made sure he left the relationship first.

If you are mentally exhausted, you may tend to look at your world from a negative perspective. Your patience for others will be low and the smallest incident can easily upset you. Being mentally exhausted can lead to errors and accidents due to poor judgements.

As you release your worries and blaming others for your current circumstance, you are creating a space for mental rest. This also ties in with having spiritual rest. If you believe in God, Source, or whatever you call as your higher power, placing your worries and your concerns on someone who is bigger than you, can lead to spiritual rest.

Whether or not you believe in or practice a religion, I believe you need to have something in your life that is outside of you to rely on. A spiritual practice is very important. When I am talking about a spiritual practice, I am not referring to attending a church, temple, or synagogue on a weekly basis as a duty. I am talking about what puts your soul at ease.

Prayer, praise and worship may be practices that can be used to release the heaviness of your spirit. Setting aside space to have quiet time or to meditate for minutes of peace. Taking a walk in a park and observing nature and listening to the birds and tree leaves rustle, may soothe your spirit.

Creating art works and music can seem like you are being a gateway of full expression of creativity. This may energize your soul. Art does not need to be confined to lines and techniques. You can go to your local arts & craft store and purchase a few supplies that interest you and start from whatever your mind thinks of first. If you are interested in drawing or painting and need a little guidance, check to see if there is an art class available in your community. In major cities, there are paint and sip classes where participants learn how to paint while they are drinking wine and socializing. If you are into fashion or design, buy items that will inspire you to create outfits, jewelry, shoes, or home accessories. You can research information on the internet or on YouTube on how to make whatever you want to make. The outcome isn't important. What is important is that you are having fun and surprising yourself of what you're capable of.

For some people, listening to their favorite music de-stresses them. Others like to create their own music. If you always wanted to learn how to play an instrument, take the opportunity to sign up for a class. Why not step out of the box and try to listen to other cultural music?

Do what will make you feel like time doesn't matter and that this one moment can stretch into eternity. That is the space where the spirit can be revitalized.

Another practice of the spirit is gratitude. Gratitude takes your mind away from looking at what should have happened in your life and what you wish would happen in the future. It places you in the current moment to be grateful for all that you have right now.

For example, Beth had a cynical view on life. Her cynicism cost her a few personal and professional relationships. Beth would like to change, but she didn't know how. She read an article about gratitude. Of course, in her mind, she had nothing to be grateful for. However, what she read in the article did not leave her mind. She decided to take the 30-day challenge of writing down three things she was grateful for at the end of the day.

The first night, she couldn't write anything down. The second night, she wrote "This is stupid." The third night, "That I get a moment to sit still and look at an empty book." The fourth night, she wrote two things, "I have a place to live" and "I have food to eat." On the fifth night, she was able to write three things down.

By the middle of the challenge, Beth started writing down more than three things and the list became less superficial. Closer to the end of the challenge, Beth started noticing the world from a different lens and began to become more optimistic in her conversations. At the end of the 30-day challenge, writing down what she was grateful for became Beth's normal routine. Her last entry for that night was, "I am grateful for the courage to take the opportunity to change even when it scared me to death."

Gratitude has a way of making you value the people, things, and opportunities that are in and will come into your life. It also reminds you how far you've come up to today and to not take anything for granted. Be grateful for this moment of now and its possibilities.

There is one spiritual practice that I believe does not get enough attention and that is kindness. As children, we are typically taught to be kind to others. If you continue to practice kindness to others, when was the last time you were kind to yourself? All of us have our critics in our heads. We can be extremely hard on ourselves. Our bodies don't look the way we would like, our hair is too this or too that, we are disappointed in ourselves for not having the talents and skills other people have, we have regrets on how we reacted to certain situations or decisions we have made. The list can go on and on.

But what if, just what if, you can take the challenge to look and treat yourself with kindness. Instead of looking at what you don't like about your body, appreciate it for being healthy.

I've always had weight issue since I was a child. I've been a size 0 – 20. I've dealt with everything from bullying to intense self-criticism of my body. In comparison to other girls that I was around, I had big thighs. I used to call them "thunder thighs." I noticed when I was in college that I tended to gain weight when I was dealing with a personal situation I couldn't resolve. As soon as that situation found its resolution, I began to lose the weight.

Because of my insecurity with my weight, I've trained myself to get ready for the day or night without looking at my body. If I did, immediately I will start picking, pulling or pinching. I always wanted to be a weight that I used to be and when I reached the weight that I wanted to be, it wasn't enough. I wanted an 8-pack.

When I made the decision to make the changes necessary to get rid of dermatographia, being self-critical, judgmental, or mean to my body was on the list for change. I made the commitment to not criticize my body or my relationship with food.

One night while standing in front of a full body mirror, I started to focus on the cellulite on my legs. After a few minutes, a thought came to me that while I was looking at what I didn't like about my legs, these legs were healthy and have walked many miles around the world. When I recognized this thought, I started to speak out loud all the great things each of my limbs has done for me and how grateful I was for that. I noticed that in that moment, I was becoming grateful to be alive and healthy with a body that has sustained me throughout my life.

When it came to food, I realized that in the times I needed comfort and no one was around, food comforted me. It helped me cope with circumstances I couldn't understand or handle. It helped me to survive the emotional, physical, and sexual traumas I've experienced by numbing me out from intolerable situations. However, I made the choice moving forward that food will not be my comfort or escapism anymore, with the exception of indulging my sugar craving once in a while, I view food as a resource for energy. I no longer allow myself to criticize me for what I am eating.

Instead of studying how your hair is not working the way you'd like, appreciate that you still have hair. For skills and talents that you don't have, what about the skills and talents you do have? To someone else, your skills and talents are needed. As for the decisions that you made and now regret, go easy on yourself. You made those decisions based on information, emotions, and choices at the time. The fact those decisions weigh heavy on your mind are reminders that you still have an opportunity to change your mind, communicate with, apologize to, or forgive others and yourself. Be kind to yourself. You've come a long way.

Using the physical, mental and spiritual tools I've suggested will help you overcome your symptoms triggers. I hope while you were reading about these tools, that you were able to think of other tools that may work for you. This will provide a sense of balance in your life. So go ahead and have the dance off with your kids, the long walk at your local park, and the spa treatment you've been desiring. Release your worry and blaming others to obtain mental rest. Give it to a power greater than you or create the space to release your soul. Finally, always show gratitude and be kind.

Chapter 6:
Finding Your Team

An old proverb says "Birds of a feather flock together." It means that individuals with similar characters or interests usually spend time together. Sometimes this saying is used when someone wants to look down or disapprove of a group of individuals. People usually judge others by who the person associates with.

The truth is that the individuals in our families, friends, work place, school, community, and who we admire in the media can have a big impact in our lives. If you are surrounded people who have a positive outlook, you will eventually start looking at your life from a positive perspective. If you are a positive person and you begin to hang around complainers, over time you will begin to start complaining. Whether you want to or not, you will begin to be influenced by others as you spend more time with them.

Have you noticed that rich people tend to be around other rich people? Mothers with small kids tend to spend time with other mothers with small children. Athletes can be seen hanging out with other athletes. Entrepreneurs have lunch meetings with other entrepreneurs. Although the old proverb can have a negative connotation, there are people who meet with others with similar interests to share or relate their experiences and interests or to be mentored.

Take a moment to think about how you act or change when you're around the circle of people in your life. In any association, the group you connect with should make you feel good being a part of it or give you a sense of family or community. In most cases, if you are around individuals that do not make you feel good or does not feel like a positive community, you have an option to leave the group of people you've associated with.

There are times when it may be difficult for someone to make the decision to walk away from their family or relationship that is not healthy. It may not be an easy decision or even be an option. I will not get into details of the reasons why someone may have a challenge to make this choice. However, if you are dealing with domestic violence, sexual abuse, or molestation, please reach out to someone you trust for help or contact an organization specialized in the abuse you are dealing with. Most organizations, like the National Domestic Violence Hotline, have toll-free numbers and a website with information that will help you identity the type of abuse you are suffering. Reach out, there is someone waiting to help you.

I would like talk about toxic relationships. Dr. Asa Don Brown defined a toxic relationship as "any relations that is unfavorable to you or others."

I believe toxic relationships can be a factor to cause symptoms of dermatographia to appear. You can have a toxic relationship with anyone – a family member, a friend, a partner, or a coworker. After a period of time, a toxic relationship can break down your spirit. Once you are mentally and spiritually worn down, your body will manifest in dis-ease.

Sometimes, someone may get into or stay in a toxic relationship because there are characteristics or actions of the other person that is familiar. There is a subconscious attraction because the person choosing the relationship had an upbringing that displayed the dynamics of a toxic relationship and consider it was normal or how love is supposed to be. Another reason someone may get into or stay in toxic relationship is because they do not believe or don't know they are worthy of a healthy relationship. Due to their low self-esteem, if this person is presented or has a chance to get into a healthier relationship, they will sabotage it because it feels foreign.

How do you know if you are in a toxic relationship? If you ever feel emotionally or psychologically stressed or drained, guarded, confused, manipulated, or unsafe when you are around or interacting with the person and boundaries are not respected, you are most likely in a toxic relationship.

Anna was in a relationship with Paul for the last five years. They had been through a lot together and were loyal to each other. Then Paul was laid off from his job from a major company. He started to look for work at other companies but was unsuccessful in being hired. Although Anna worked a full-time job, without Paul working, their savings would be depleted in a couple of weeks.

Anna began to notice when she arrived home from work that Paul would begin to talk down to her. He would speak negatively about her cooking. When Anna tried to share a bad experience at work, Paul would tell her that what she was going through was nothing compared to him. He hadn't been able to get a job for the last three months. Occasionally, Paul would make snide remarks to Anna. She would tell herself that he would change once he was able to find work. Now, Anna was trying to spend more time at work or socializing with friends to avoid feeling stress or drained by Paul's presence. They had been through a lot, but his constant verbal attacks were wearing her down psychologically.

The best way to get out of a toxic relationship is to first acknowledge you are in one, if that is the case. Since such a relationship can cause you to doubt yourself and help create or increase low self-esteem, I would suggest that you reach out for professional help. You can reach out to a licensed therapist, psychologist or a respected minister in your place of worship.

As you are working through this transition with professional help and begin to have revelation of a healthier lifestyle, you will learn and become aware of boundaries. You will realize that you are not willing to go back to the lifestyle you use to live. This is a good time to start developing new positive relationships and find your team.

When you are looking for new associates, friends, or community for your team, create a checklist of what type of characteristic you would like to have in these new relationships. Pick characteristics that will support and encourage you through your transition. Look for people who want only the best for you, who enjoy your company and you like theirs. Try to find someone you can learn from, someone you can teach, someone you can have fun with and relax, someone who shares your passion of your interest, someone who can check you, if needed and another person who will encourage you. If you have a close friend or family member who have been with you through your ups and downs, if they are still available, put them on your team. Your team is collection of individuals who see past your struggles and mistakes and accept you as you are.

Wouldn't it be nice to have a makeup artist, hairdresser, fashion stylist and gym trainer ready to get you picture perfect for the camera like celebrities do? Well, you can. It may not be at the level of celebrities or your favorite reality star, but you can create your own style team.

The people who are currently providing you professional services are a part of your team. If you like the styles your hairdresser or barber creates, they are on your team. If you can afford it, you can hire a personal trainer at your local gym to help you get in shape. If you can't afford a personal trainer, join an exercise group and act as though the instructor is your trainer. The personal trainer or the instructor are a part of your team.

If you need to update or upgrade your fashion style, there a few popular department stores who offer personal shopping services. If the personal shopping service is not available, you can ask a fashion savvy friend if she or he would like to spend the day with you shopping and you will buy them lunch or dinner for their time. Add them to the team. If you want your make-up done or want to know what skin care will work for you, there are many make-up or skin stores, that will offer free make-up sessions or skin care consultations when you make a small purchase. The other option is to visit a local beauty school and see if their students offer make-up services at a reasonable price. The artist or the consultant is on your team.

Now none of these individuals need to know they are on your "team." However, just like celebrities, you are paying them to help you look your best. It is another way to feel supported as you become the person you want to be without being concerned about dermatographia.

Chapter 7:
Enough is Enough

Have you ever heard some say, "Enough is enough?" That person was probably sick and tired of dealing with whatever they were talking about and wanted it to stop. In their situation, boundaries were crossed. Boundaries are necessary to establish your identity. If you do not set boundaries, you will begin to feel anger and resentment toward others. This can also lead to depression and burnout. Boundaries keep us safe and are important for self-care.

What is self-care? On her website moneycrashers.com, Mary McCoy describes self-care as a "very active and powerful choice to engage in the activities that are required to gain or maintain an optimal level of overall health. And in this case, overall health includes not just the physical, but the psychological, emotional, social, and spiritual components of an individual's well-being."

If we are lacking boundaries in one area in our life, it will cause a domino effect in other areas. Here are some examples of lack of boundaries:

1. You've put in long hours at work, you're tired, everyone has gone home, and you're done for the day. As you are getting ready to walk out the door, your boss comes in and asks if you are leaving. You tell your boss "yes" as you turn back to the door. Then your boss starts talking to you about an upcoming project. You do not leave the office until an hour later.

2. Your mother comes to your place to visit for a couple of weeks. While you are more than accommodating to her and show her great hospitality, every other day she is asking you to take her to the store, so she can buy something.

3. You are visiting a good friend of yours at lunch. You enjoy spending time with her. The only issue is that she talks badly about a mutual friend of yours. In the past, you've asked her not to talk about this person with you. When you see your friend at the restaurant, you're having a great time, and everything goes smoothly. Then your friend tells you, "I know you told me that you don't want me to talk about this person, but…"

4. You have a deadline by tomorrow morning. It's lunch time and you're hungry. You tell yourself, let me just finish a little bit more then I will go eat. You keep telling yourself this until you can't concentrate anymore. You look at the clock and it's time for you to leave. As you are leaving the parking lot, you snap at the parking attendant for being too slow.

5. You and your co-worker go out for happy hour at a nearby restaurant. You know your limit is two drinks. After you've had your two drinks, a couple of your co-workers pressure you into having two more drinks. The next morning you are regretting it and feel upset with yourself.

6. To feel sane throughout the day, you have learned that you need to meditate for a few minutes in the morning before you start your day. Recently, your schedule is packed more than usual. Now whenever you get up, you get ready for the day and leave your place without meditating. Lately, you've been short with people and feel worn down.

7. When your spouse is frustrated, she tends to talk to you in a condescending way that makes you feel small. You have asked her to stop, and she slowed it down, but every once in a while, a comment or two will slip out.

So, let go over these examples and talk about the boundaries crossed, what aspect of the overall health is being impacted and a possible response.

1. The boss has crossed a boundary by not respecting that it is time for you to leave to go home. You may appreciate that you are being respected, but you may feel stuck from leaving, because it's your boss. This can impact your psychological well-being.

   Possible response: "Mr./Ms.___, I am really interested in talking about the project, is it late and I would like to go home. Is it possible that we schedule some time together tomorrow morning and continue this conversation?"

2. In this example, your mother's action says that she does not respect your time. This can impact your emotional well-being.

   Possible response: "Hi mom, can you make a list of all of the items you need and places you would like to go to? I have Friday off and I would like to make the time for you to run your errands."

3. Although you've already set your boundary with your friend, it seems like she is not taking you seriously. This can impact your social well-being.

   Possible response: "_____, before you go any further, I've already shared with you my feelings about talking about our friend. I am asking you again to respect my request. Let's talk about dessert instead."

4. This example is when you cross a boundary with yourself. Your body is hungry, and you are making work a priority over your health. This can impact your physical well-being.

   Possible response: "I need to stop right now and get something to eat. If I don't I am going to hangry and bite someone's head off."

5. Example five is similar to four. You knew your limit, but you ignored your conscious to succumb to the pressure to be accepted by your peers. This can impact your physical, psychological and social well-being.

   Possible response: "You know what guys, I would like to continue with you, but I've reached my limit. Anyway, it is time for me to go. It was a pleasure spending time with you."

6. This is another example of not respecting yourself. This will impact you spiritual well-being.

   Possible response: Take a deep breath before you open the door to leave. Remind yourself it is only a few minutes that can balance your whole day. If you must, meditate for less time, so you can be centered.

7. You've set your boundary with your spouse, but she stills sneaks in her remarks. This will impact your psychological and emotional well-being.

   Possible response: Do this in the spirit of love. "Honey, I've asked you before not to talk to me in a condescending manner, when you talk to me in that tone it makes me feel small and not valued. I am asking you again to please stop."

As you set boundaries, it is also a way of saying "no." Saying "no" can be a challenge for some people. If we don't learn how to say "no" to things that do not allow us to be comfortable in our skin and around others, we are essentially allowing people to take advantage of us with our permission.

While you are establishing your identity, you will learn what makes you feel comfortable, appreciated, respected, and safe and what does not. When you begin to set your boundaries, it will feel uncomfortable, almost wrong. You may begin to wonder if you should have said what you said or if you were a little harsh. As you continue, it will get easier. You will know when it becomes your normal, when you do not set up a boundary with someone or yourself, and you feel like you've betrayed your spirit.

When you are setting a boundary:

1. **Learn your comfort zone, what you will permit or will not allow.**

This is your "do not cross this line" zone or your deal breakers.

2. **Recognize your limits.**

    You know what you can offer without over-extending yourself. Pay attention to your body and intuition for signals for what will not work for you.

3. **Know you have a right to say "No."**

    You can tell someone no without any explanation or guilt.

4. **Assertively inform the person what you expect them from them or what you won't do.**

    You do not need to be rude or disrespectful when you are setting your boundary. When you place firm guidelines, you will be taken seriously.

5. **Stick to what you've said.**

    There will be people who will challenge your boundaries, like the friend at lunch example.

6. **Have an exit strategy.**

    Be prepared for someone to ignore everything you said. If this happens, the person does not respect you at all. It's time to exit.

7. **Let go of the outcome.**

    When you start practicing boundaries it will ruffle some major feathers. Let it go. This is about and for you.

8. **Be proud of yourself that you have you as a priority.**
   You've come a long way to get to this point. You are showing yourself that you are worth the space that you need to be at peace and be present for what matters to you.

Boundaries are not about isolating yourself, or not wanting to be helpful or a team player. It's about limits to keep you safe and healthy so you can be there for others when needed. To overcome dermatographia, it is important to set boundaries so you can put your health first.

Chapter 8:

This Way, Please

We are going to talk about what really matters and the importance of practicing to avoid reoccurring symptoms of dermatographia. What you think, what you say, your environment, taking responsibility, and letting go of baggage play a significant role in the process. It is like a house. We've set the foundation with the prior chapters. Now we have put the walls up, then place the windows in and attach the roof. I will also add what I believe is the secret to avoiding future outbreaks of dermatographia.

The first thing that matters is our thoughts. Our thoughts can change the course of our lives. How we think creates the view of how we look at our surroundings. If we think the sky is blue, then no matter how gray it is, we will believe the sky is blue. If you think Mondays suck, then Mondays suck. As we think we can make a sale, then we can make sale.

As we continue to think about the things and circumstances that we want, and we start to see their manifestations, then our thoughts become beliefs. Our beliefs are collections of experiences that we can trust and rely on. They can us help achieve our goals or hold us back from growing. We use our beliefs as guides of truth to walk through our life.

Dealing with dermatographia, there is a lot that you have to focus on. We already went over triggers, symptoms, deciding to change your life, tools you need to practice, creating your team and setting boundaries. That's a lot to think about at one time. You may think, "How can I do all of this?" You can by starting with and focusing on one thing at a time. Remember, I mentioned all you need is to decide to be committed. Think about your commitment. Remind yourself on why you decided to make a change.

Roger learned his triggers for his dermatographia and began to practice his new spiritual tool of gratitude. He felt the need to move forward in the process, and at the same time he wanted to start exercising at the gym. Roger had a very tight traveling schedule in the upcoming few months. When he arrived at the destination, he usually had to deal with jet lag. He felt too tired to work out like he planned. Roger decided to focus on getting rest and continue with his gratitude journal.

When you are reminded of your commitment, you will hold yourself accountable to finish what you started. If challenges arise, you can think about how much you've accomplished. Having positive and encouraging thoughts will be the drive to push you forward. Being present to recognize this will help you keep moving forward. This is a practice.

The second thing that matters is what you say. Words matter. Usually when we tell someone we are going to do something for them, they will wait in expectation for it to be completed. If it is not completed as expected, we lose credibility because we did not keep our word. Words can make an impact on our relationships, work environment, and ourselves.

Words are powerful. You can share with someone encouraging words and it can brighten up their day. The words you speak out in anger will have another person mirror your emotions. What you say to others can change the atmosphere in a room.

There are times, when it is best not to say anything at all. It could be because what you're going through is nobody's business. It could also be that you may not have someone you can trust to keep what you have to say in confidence. You might not say anything to anyone because you may not be able to articulate your thoughts, or you want to do something as a surprise. You may not speak to certain people about your experiences because you may be ridiculed.

Daniella was recently diagnosed with dermatographia. She usually had her outbreak on her chest and legs. She hadn't shared the news with anyone in her family. Daniella was planning on attending a family get-together that weekend. She wore a top with sleeves to her elbows. During dinner, someone accidentally scratched Daniella. Daniella didn't think anything about it until an aunt asked what happened to her arm. Daniella looked down and saw a large welt there. When everyone at the dinner turned to look at Daniella, she said that it was nothing, just a small scratch. Thirty minutes later, the same aunt said that for such a small scratch there was a very large welt. Someone else asked Daniella if she was okay. Daniella began to feel self-conscious and uncomfortable at the dinner. She asked a cousin for a sweater to put on to avoid any additional attention.

Dealing with dermatographia is a challenge. A lot of people have not heard of dermatographia. It is not a popular skin condition. If you want to share your experience with dermatographia, make sure it is with people who are open to understanding the condition. If you would like to share your experience with the exercises in this book and how it is helping you overcome dermatographia, do it with people who are encouraging and supportive. Their positive feedback will encourage you in return.

Have you paid attention to how you speak to yourself? If so, is it positive or negative?

The same way your words have an impact on others, it can have an impact on you. Your thoughts about dermatographia is your internal dialogue. Although you may not speak the words out loud, your internal dialogue is still speaking to you, impacting your health in a positive or negative way. Practice to guard what you say to yourself.

The third thing that matters is how you see your world. Your perspective about your past and others will make a big impact on your dermatographia symptoms. No one's life is perfect. We've all suffered from pain, loss, betrayal, rejection, abandonment, or trauma at some time in our life. The healing process may take a lifetime to be completed.

When we look at our past, we are reminded of our suffering and what we feel like we miss out on. This is a holdout of unforgiveness. If you keep looking back at what should have been, could have happened, would have received, you are holding yourself hostage in that time period. You will not be able to appreciate what you have in the present and really know where you are going in the future, because you are stuck. The feeling of being stuck comes from not releasing your judgments from the past.

To help you release yourself from being stuck, I have an exercise that I would like you to try. Think of a memory in your past that was not comfortable or was embarrassing. Make sure you do not use this exercise with traumatic or intense memories, if you are not in the presence of a professional.

For example, you had an instructor who told his class that he would not allow any late students to enter his class once he started teaching. One day, you were rushing to class and you showed up late after he started teaching. The instructor stopped teaching, looked at you and made an example of you in front of the class and then told you to leave.

After you have your unpleasant memory, I would like you to think about a positive outcome that came out of that experience.

For example, since the incident with your instructor, you are always five minutes early to every event and you respect people's time.

As you practice this exercise, you will become aware of the positive traits, skills and characteristics that you earn from your past experiences. You will start to notice that you have more in and around you than you thought.

Finally, your environment matters. Create a sacred space that is quiet and just for you. This sacred space may be your home, a room, a closet or your car. This is an area where you can be completely yourself. You can let yourself go and do a little crazy dance if you want to. This space is your safe zone. The safe zone allows you not only to be silly, it permits you to express your emotions out loud freely without judgement. When we keep all our emotions inside our bodies, our body starts to manifest our emotions into illnesses. You need give yourself permission to release your emotions, so you can process your pain and heal.

Rhonda was a single mother of two boys. She worked a full-time job and attended college part-time. She and her family lived in a two-story home, and underneath the stairs was a storage room. Rhonda had converted the storage room into her sacred space. She added items into the room that made her feel safe and comfortable. She changed the door and added a lock to prevent her children from going into the room to play. After her children were in bed, Rhonda went into her sacred space to meditate, pray, cry, or just to enjoy the peace and quiet. The time she spent in her room allowed her to think, relax, process her day, or plan for the future.

Many of us have had traumatic experiences, yet we survived it. Whatever coping mechanism was used to get to this very day was necessary for our survival. However, there comes a point when our coping devices no longer work. This leads to taking responsibility.

Taking responsibility is the awareness and acknowledging that what worked for you in the past no longer serves you in the present and is keeping you back from your future. It is being mindful that you cannot move forward into the life you desire if you are still holding onto the pain of your past, which I refer to as baggage. It is also knowing that you are tired of your victim mentality and you cannot go through the next phase in your life without help. It is the desire to make a change.

If you are currently suffering from your traumatic experience, again I would suggest that you seek professional help to process your pain. If you are not comfortable seeing a psychologist or a licensed therapist, talk to a trusted minister or mentor. Coming face to face with the truth versus your story is challenging and can be emotional. However, when you've overcome the emotional pain and begin the healing process, you will be able to reassess where you are in your life right now from a healthier perspective.

If you've overcome a childhood trauma, a question you may ask yourself is "As an adult, how can I take action to do things differently?" or "What can I do as an adult that will show me that I am not a victim to my past?". If you've overcome a trauma as an adult, a question you may ask is, "What can I do to show to myself that I've taken back my power?" or "How can I help or serve others who have suffered what I've overcome and become a light of hope for them?" These types of questions will lead to actions. When you take responsibility, you stand in your own authority and take back your power to not allow your past to control your life anymore.

David came home after his final tour in Afghanistan. He was diagnosed with Post Traumatic Stress Disorder (PTSD). He was offered an opportunity to see a psychologist but turned it down. After a few months, David realized that he couldn't seem to function in the way that he wanted. His life at home seemed alien to him compared to the war that he left behind. He decided to see the psychologist.

After a year and a half of therapy, David was beginning to get adjusted to normal life. He began to think of ways he could help other active duty military members who suffered from PTSD and struggled with acclimating to their old routines at home. David found a local organization that served active duty military personnel and veterans who suffered from PTSD. He volunteered at the organization every week while he continued his therapy.

Soon David was asked to share his story at various community centers throughout the city. As time passed, David began to feel like his life was no longer controlled by PTSD. He began to make new connections with other organizations that showed interest in his story. The speaking events began to give David a sense of purpose. The greatest gift that David received was when someone approached him and told him how much his story had changed their life.

Everyone's process and timetable to healing is different. For some it may take months and years, or a lifetime for others. Healing is not a competition or an item to check off your list. It is continuous in one form or another. When you take the actions to release yourself from the bondage of your past, the weight, the baggage of your pain will start to diminish or is eliminated. You will find new energy to focus on what you've been wanting to do. As you continue on in your healing journey, you may find out new things about yourself that you did not know you were capable of or had an interest in. The future now seems full of potential, promise and excitement.

There is one thing that I believe is the secret of me overcoming dermatographia. It is finding and doing things that bring me joy. I am referring to activities that makes me feel excited like a little child, spurs creativity, gives me the desire to do it all the time and I feel contentment. As a boundary, I do not participate in activities that do not fall in one of those categories.

Notice that I did not mention "things that make me happy." Happiness is relative. With happiness, I am working on an activity and if it doesn't work out like I wanted it to, then I am no longer happy. Doing things with joy comes from within. It doesn't matter about the outcome. What matters is the moment in the activity.

Here is another exercise for you. Can you list at least three things that bring you joy?

If you are not able to complete the list, think about what you did as a child that made you joyful. You can also think about activities that you've been curious about and have yet to try. Is there an activity you used to do as an adult, that you stopped doing because life got in the way?

Try to think up five things that will bring you joy. Test them out to see if they are still the right fit for you. When you find your top three, start participating in those activities regularly. These "bring you joy" activities will take your mind off your dermatographia and help you start living your life to the fullest.

I've provided you with five traits and one secret that will help you gain control over dermatographia. You have an opportunity to practice them and do the exercises as often as you like. As you practice these traits, you will notice that your mindset will begin to change to a positive outlook.

Chapter 9:

Rewind

By now, you have come a long way. You're been steadily practicing your tools, and you're comfortable with your team. You confidently set your boundaries to maintain your overall health, you are conscious of your thoughts and actions, and guard your sacred space. Life seems to be going smoothly and you haven't felt this good in a while, or ever. You are now entertaining your stagnant dreams, or you are actively pursuing them.

Then when you least expect it – a break-up, a loss of a family member, a job or promotion loss, a divorce, an illness, or anything else you may have not seen coming. Any of these situations can be difficult for anyone, but it may feel like a whirlwind to you. During this time, you may feel stunned. Thinking about your process is way in the back of your mind.

How you deal with the situation may be different for each person. You may have stayed so committed to everything you have practiced that it has become your normal lifestyle, or you've realized that somehow you've stopped using every tool that you started with. Maybe you've held on to one practice, but it feels like you've fallen off the wagon. You've probably stopped contacting the close members of you team. Boundaries and sacred space? Barely holding on to the skeleton of what you knew. Whether you stayed committed despite everything that is going on or you dropped the ball; the stress is unbearable.

The itchiness and the symptoms have reappeared. You have gone back to ask the same questions you asked when dermatographia first started showing up. You feel lost and confused. You may ask, "How did I get here?", "Why is this showing up again?", or "I thought I got rid of this?" What you are experiencing is a relapse.

When you are under extreme stress, not matter how diligent you've been, there is a possibility of having a relapse. No one wants to know or feel like they are going backwards. Especially after investing so much time, effort, and money to get better. The feelings you can experience are disappointment, sadness, and may be feel like a failure.

This does not prove that you have failed at accomplishing your dream. New challenges or obstacles are like tests. No one likes taking tests. Before you take a test, you learn the material, and then you take one or two practice quizzes. Once you know the date of the test, you may be someone who sets aside time to study or likes to cram the night before.

You hope the test questions would be like past quizzes and something you can quickly recognize. But when you get the test, it looks nothing like you've expected. It's the right topic, the questions are in a standard format, the way the questions are worded tells you that this test is not going to be easy. Just because the way the questions are worded are not as you expected, does not mean that you do not know the material.

When you are faced with a new challenge or obstacle, you are surprised because the content and the timing of the circumstance and don't meet your expectations. Once you get the chance to step back and look at where you are, you can evaluate the situation from a different perspective. You will be able to shift around how you react, to suit the state that you are in.

If you stopped using all the tools, because it became too much to handle, it's okay. Find one tool you can continue and modify it. For example, maybe you used to take an hour walk in the morning, which gave you peace and allowed you to think clearly. Now you're in an environment where a park is not available, and you don't have time to walk in the mornings. Could you walk around the neighborhood for 15 – 20 minutes before sunset?

Another example is not being able to continue an activity that used to bring you joy, like playing a sport, due to your finances. Try to look for free opportunities to continue the activity at community centers, churches or volunteer to teach others what you've learned of from your sport.

When you are challenged to do something that is out of your norm, create new or adjust your methods of your daily practice. There will be times when you can use one tool out of your toolbox and it will be your saving grace. Be creative. You know your stuff. Trust yourself to make the best decisions for your benefit.

Being aware of relapses or setbacks, are a part of the journey. Don't be too hard on yourself if this occurs to you. You do not have to go through this trial with perfect scores and it is not timed. Just take it slow until you have an opportunity to jump right back in the game.

Chapter 10:
Conclusion

Let's recap everything we've gone over. We've identified dermatographia, its symptoms, and your possible reaction to your symptoms. We went over the emotional toll dermatographia may cause and the fears you may face while you're having dermatographia episodes. You were able to recognize the costs of living with dermatographia and its impact on your finances, relationships, confidence, and body.

I shared my journey with symptoms of severe dermatographia until I received a diagnosis. This diagnosis became the defining moment for me to make dramatic changes in my life. I also explained the process that I took to live my life until I was able to live without any outbreaks of dermatographia.

You've learned the possible triggers for your symptoms, acknowledged the triggers, and made the decision to make a change. You were provided physical, mental, and spiritual tools which you can practice daily. These tools are intended to provide you a sense of balance in your life.

We discussed how the people in your life can influence you in a positive or negative way and that everyone tends to associate with others that have common interests. We talked about toxic relationships and when it is time to get professional help. As you begin to create your new identity, you will start to set boundaries and develop new relationship with people who become your team.

You learned how to set boundaries with family, friends, work, and yourself and you realized that you need to continue to practice the tools consistently to avoid causing a reoccurrence of symptoms. As you navigate through this journey, you understand that you will have to continue to work on how you think about yourself and others. That you need to maintain a positive mindset. As you make changes, your environment will change around you.

At the end of it, when life throws you a surprise and knocks you off guard, you can suffer a relapse. It may seem like everything you worked for was for nothing. However, the tools that you've received don't go away because life happens. You just have use what you know in a different way.

It was my goal for this book to share what I've learned in my journey to live my life free from dermatographia. I've listed major contributors to what created my symptoms and how I've overcome my symptoms. As you were reading any of the chapters, if you have different or additional triggers and symptoms, let's acknowledge them. If you thought of new tools or solutions, go ahead and use them. Use what works for you but go through the process.

Can I be real with you? This process is not an overnight fix. As I shared in my story, it took two years for the symptoms of dermatographia to stop all together. Although, I don't have to worry about dermatographia, I still have the scars as a reminder of my outbreaks. As stated, there will be accomplishments and setbacks, but you have everything you need to make this happen. This is very important to keep in mind. So, as you go through this journey, please be patient and kind to yourself. I believe that you can make your dream come true.

However, if you want to want to accomplish your dream life of living freely without being concerned or affected by dermatographia, don't hesitate to contact me. I know the process will be faster, easier and you would more likely succeed if we work together. I look forward and would be excited to be a part of your team.

If you would like to share your success story or have questions, you can contact me by email at sandra@sandragraneau.com. I look forward to hearing from you.

Blessings!

Acknowledgments

I want to say thank you to my family who loved me when I didn't feel lovable and believe that I am still capable of anything, even when I've changed my mind for the 100th time.

To the Morgan James Publishing team: Special thanks to David Hancock, CEO & Founder for believing in me and my message. To my Author Relations Manager, Gayle West, thanks for making the process seamless and easy. Many more thanks to everyone else, but especially Jim Howard, Bethany Marshall, and Nickcole Watkins.

There are people who became family even though they are not related by blood. To the Lawhorn, Linares, and Ahmad families, no matter how far I am away, when I return you've always welcomed me back with open arms.

This book wouldn't have happened if it wasn't for Cathy S. Harris, LCSW who challenged me to start writing books to tell my story to help others.

I want to say thank you to my life coach instructors from Life Purpose Institute – Diana Long, Tanya Mundo, and Gretchen Hydo. All of you set a standard and a space for growth that I would like to exemplify for my coaching clients.

To Terry Ross, I am so grateful that I took a leap into acting with you as my guide.

To those of you who are on my team to help get me healthy, relaxed and beautiful, you are appreciated.

To my friends who have been with me through my worst and my best, and still want to hang out. I am so grateful to you. "Where do you want to eat?"

This book was only completed by the grace of God. For that no words can be expressed.

About the Author

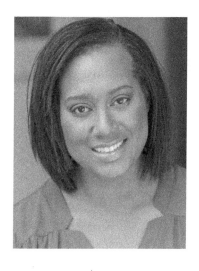

Originally from the beautiful U.S. Virgin Islands, Sandra spent her childhood in San Diego, CA and her teen years in St. Thomas, U.S.V.I. She returned to Southern California for college and earned her B.S. in management from California State University, Northridge.

After college, Sandra spent ten years in management positions for several companies. The long hours took their toll on her body and it wasn't until she was diagnosed with dermatographia that she realized that she needed to make a significant change in the way she was living her life.

When she finally made the decision to act on the things her heart was calling her to do, her life slowly began to transition into the life of her dreams. She enrolled at the Life Purpose Institute in San Diego, CA and earned her Professional Certified Coach Certificate. She also started acting and fashion design as creative outlets. All the dreams that had remained dormant, Sandra is now on a mission to make come true.

She has a saying: "Don't give up on your dream(s), if your dream(s) hasn't given up on you." This is about having dreams, that she thought she was too late, too old, or too____ to be accomplished. If the dream still comes to mind, there is still time to make it happen.

Sandra is passionate about helping others live the life their heart wants them to live without any guilt, shame and judgements.

Sandra currently resides in Houston, TX. She enjoys eating out with friends, spending time with her family, looks forward to spa days, and loves to travel.

Email: sandra@sandragraneau.com

Thank You!

Hey you! Thank you for taking the time to pick up and read this book. The fact that you've gotten to this point in the book tells me something about you: you're ready. You are ready to rewrite your life story. You're ready to live your life freely without being affected by dermatographia.

If you would like to continue working with me, you can reach me by email at sandra@sandragraneau.com or visit my website at www.sandragraneau.com to schedule a *free* 30-minute strategy session. I am excited to hear from you.

CPSIA information can be obtained
at www.ICGtesting.com
Printed in the USA
LVHW090227131119
637202LV00001B/132/P